YOUR
BODY ON
SALT

BY YVETTE LaPIERRE

CONTENT CONSULTANT
Debbie Fetter, PhD
Lecturer (PSOE), Department of Nutrition
University of California, Davis

Cover image: Salt enhances the flavors of many foods, including pretzels.

Core Library

An Imprint of Abdo Publishing
abdobooks.com

abdocorelibrary.com

Published by Abdo Publishing, a division of ABDO, PO Box 398166, Minneapolis, Minnesota 55439. Copyright © 2020 by Abdo Consulting Group, Inc. International copyrights reserved in all countries. No part of this book may be reproduced in any form without written permission from the publisher. Core Library™ is a trademark and logo of Abdo Publishing.

Printed in the United States of America, North Mankato, Minnesota
022019
092019

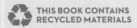

Cover Photo: Marie C. Fields/Shutterstock Images
Interior Photos: Marie C. Fields/Shutterstock Images, 1; Shutterstock Images, 4–5, 8, 14, 21, 27 (kidneys), 27 (brain), 28, 35, 45; Anthony Berenyi/Shutterstock Images, 10; Kuttelvaserova Stuchelova/Shutterstock Images, 12–13, 43; iStockphoto, 18–19; Lunasee Studios/Shutterstock Images, 22; Miro Novak/Shutterstock Images, 24–25; Puwadol Jaturawutthichai/Shutterstock Images, 30; Alexey Lysenko/Shutterstock Images, 32–33; Sheila Fitzgerald/Shutterstock Images, 36; Red Line Editorial, 39; Monkey Business Images/Shutterstock Images, 40

Editor: Marie Pearson
Series Designer: Claire Vanden Branden

Library of Congress Control Number: 2018965968

Publisher's Cataloging-in-Publication Data

Names: LaPierre, Yvette, author.
Title: Your body on salt / by Yvette LaPierre
Description: Minneapolis, Minnesota: Abdo Publishing, 2020 | Series: Nutrition and your body | Includes online resources and index.
Identifiers: ISBN 9781532118869 (lib. bdg.) | ISBN 9781532173042 (ebook) | ISBN 9781644940778 (pbk.)
Subjects: LCSH: Salt--Physiological effect--Juvenile literature. | Salt in the body--Juvenile literature. | Food--Health aspects--Juvenile literature.
Classification: DDC 613.20--dc23

CONTENTS

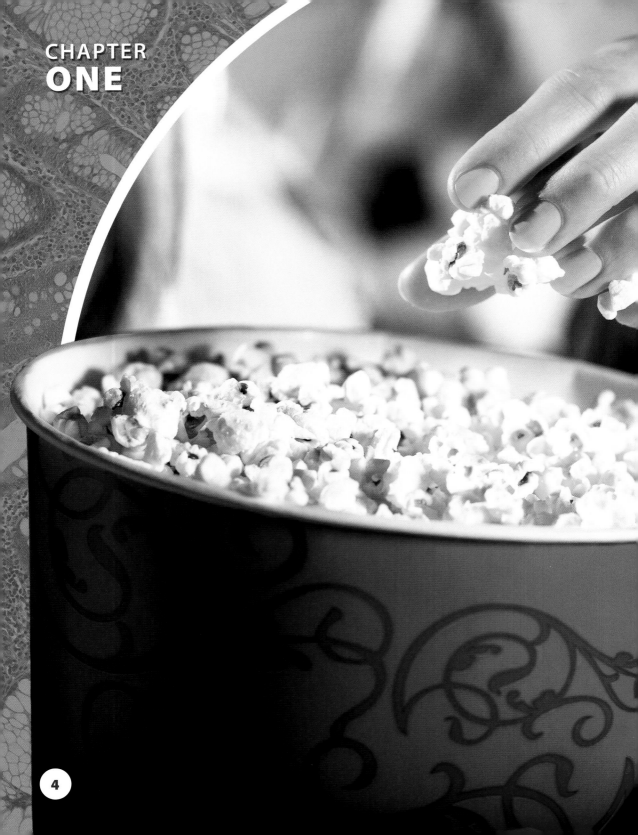

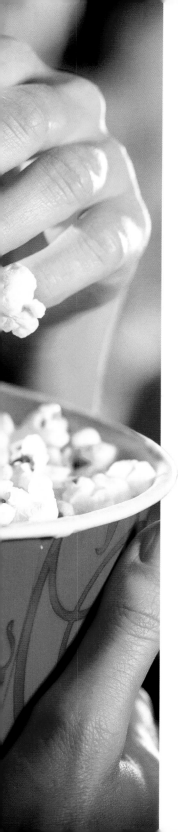

A SALTY SUBJECT

The lights dim in the movie theater. The movie starts. Jillian begins munching on her popcorn. She licks the extra salt from her fingers. Halfway through the bucket, she realizes she is thirsty. She reaches for her bottle of water and takes a big drink.

Jillian's body responds to all the salt she's eaten. The salt passes through the wall of her small intestine. It enters her bloodstream. Soon she has more salt in her blood and body fluids than in her cells. Her body senses the increase in salt and works hard to return the salt to normal levels. More water is needed to dilute the salt. Water is pulled from the body's cells

Popcorn is often made with salt and butter.

5

DOES SALT MAKE YOU THIRSTY?

Scientists used to think that when people eat a lot of salt, they get thirsty. That's been the theory for decades. But there may be more to the story, according to a 2017 study. Researchers fed two groups of men identical diets. But researchers changed the level of salt in the food. When the men ate more salt, they drank less. The extra sodium may have triggered their bodies to conserve water. They were less thirsty, not more. The study has caused scientists to rethink how the body balances salt and water.

into the body fluids. Sensors in Jillian's brain tell her she's thirsty, so she drinks more water. Balance is restored.

SALT OR SODIUM?

Many people use the terms *salt* and *sodium* interchangeably. But they are different. Salt is a natural mineral. A mineral is a substance found in the earth that does not come from a plant or animal. Salt is composed of two elements. The elements are sodium and chloride. Sodium's chemical symbol is Na. Chloride's is Cl.

Chloride is a form of chlorine. The chemical name of salt is sodium chloride, or NaCl for short.

Approximately 60 percent of salt is chloride. Only 40 percent is sodium. But when it comes to health, sodium can play a large role.

AN EDIBLE ROCK

NaCl is a rock. It's the only rock that humans eat. It dissolves in water. Most of the salt we eat comes from oceans or deep in the earth. Underground salt is mined. Salt from oceans is produced through evaporation. Canals divert seawater into shallow ponds. The water slowly dries up. Salt is left behind and gathered. Every year, people around the world consume approximately 187 million short tons (170 metric tons) of salt.

SALTY BODIES

If you lick your upper lip after sweating, it tastes salty. That's because sweat contains chloride and sodium. An average adult's body has approximately 3.5 ounces (100 grams) of sodium. That's enough to fill a salt

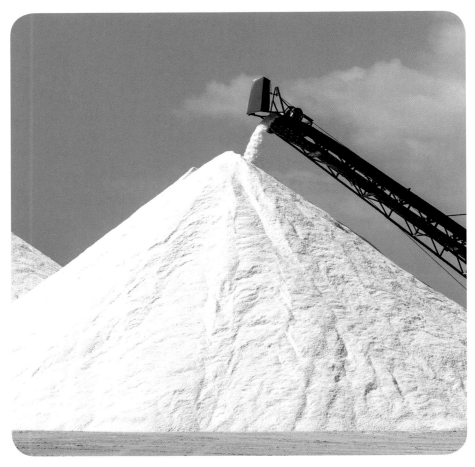

Mining companies bring underground salt to the surface to prepare for sale.

shaker or two. Blood and the fluids around body cells contain sodium.

Our bodies can't make sodium. We get it from foods and drinks. We constantly lose sodium when we cry, sweat, or go to the bathroom. We must replace the sodium by eating salt.

AN ESSENTIAL NUTRIENT

There are some nutrients the body needs but can't make or can't make enough of to meet its needs. These are called essential nutrients. Sodium is an essential nutrient. Sodium is also a micronutrient. The body only needs a small amount of it to work. But within this category, sodium is a major mineral. That means the body

SALT IN HISTORY

Salt has always been a part of human diets. Humans have sprinkled salt on food for thousands of years. People also used salt to preserve food before refrigeration. Salt is cheap and easy to get today. But that wasn't always the case. In earlier times, salt was hard to find. Collecting it was hard work. That made it expensive. Salt was so valuable that ancient Greeks used it as money. The word *salary* is from the Latin word for *salt*. Even now, people say someone is "worth his or her salt" as a compliment.

Amount Per Serving	Mix	Prepared
Calories	260	360
Calories from Fat	80	150
	% Daily Value*	
Total Fat 9g*	**14%**	**26%**
Saturated Fat 3.5g	**18%**	**30%**
Cholesterol 0mg	**0%**	**1%**
Sodium 360mg	**15%**	**20%**
Total Carbohydrate 46g	**15%**	**16%**
Dietary Fiber 1g	**4%**	**4%**
Sugars 28g		
Protein 2g		

Different foods have different levels of sodium.

needs relatively large amounts of it compared with other micronutrients.

Sodium helps keep body fluids in balance. Body fluids move nutrients and oxygen around the body and into the brain. Sodium helps keep the muscles working, including the heart. The chloride in salt is helpful too.

It helps the body balance electrolytes. Electrolytes are minerals. Chloride itself is an electrolyte.

Sometimes people have too little sodium in their bodies. That's called hyponatremia. Low sodium can be very dangerous. But most people in the United States get too much sodium. This can lead to hypernatremia, which has been linked to several health problems.

The key is to eat salt, but not too much. This will keep sodium and fluid levels in balance. That allows the body to function at its best.

EXPLORE ONLINE

Chapter One briefly discusses why our bodies need salt. It explains how the body keeps sodium levels in balance. The website below tells one way the body gets rid of excess sodium. As you know, every source is different. How is the information given in the video the same as information in this chapter? What information is different? What new information did you learn?

WONDEROPOLIS: WHY IS SWEAT SALTY?
abdocorelibrary.com/salt

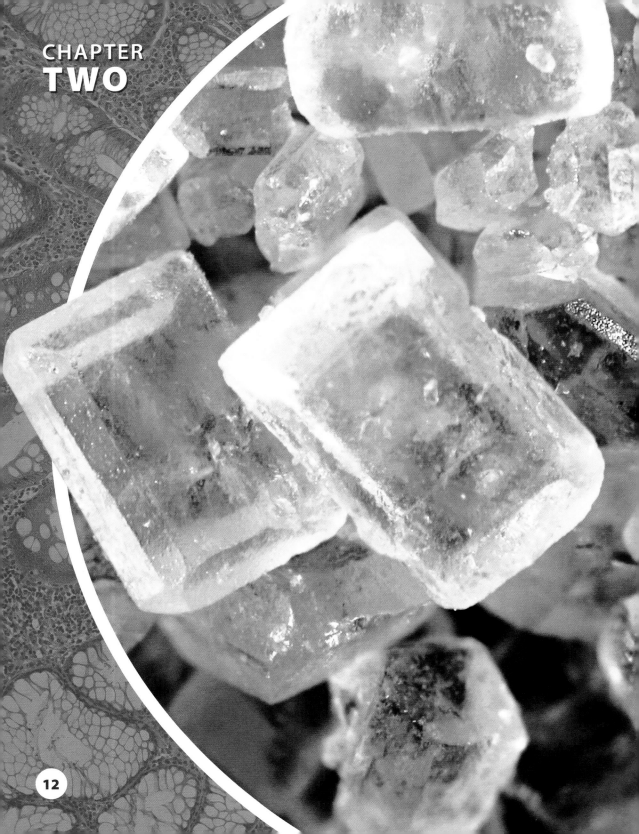

CHAPTER
TWO

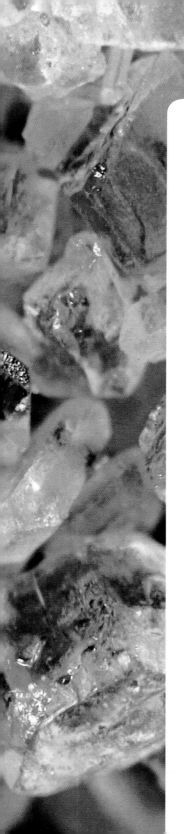

HOW SALT FUNCTIONS

The sodium and chloride in salt are electrolytes. They dissolve in body fluids. They become ions. Ions are electrically charged particles. They carry positive or negative charges. They conduct electrical impulses in the body.

Ions carry messages from the brain to the nerves and muscles. Sodium ions tell the muscles to move. They have a role in a person's senses. Senses include taste, smell, and touch. The messages also influence thirst. Electrolytes help make sure people drink enough water.

Salt forms in cube-like crystals.

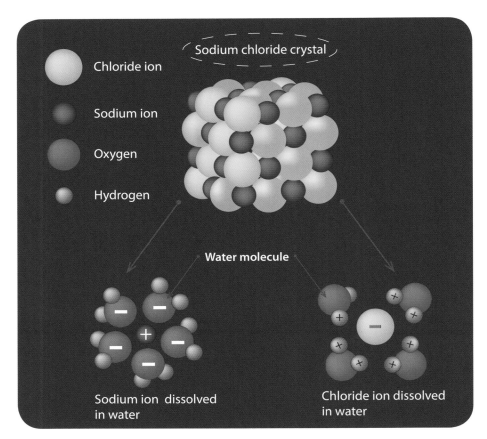

A salt crystal is made of sodium ions and chloride. When salt dissolves in water, sodium ions attract the oxygen part of a water molecule, and chloride ions attract the hydrogen parts of a water molecule.

KEEPING THE BALANCE

Salt helps keep our fluid levels in balance. Water makes up more than half of the body's weight. Water is kept in three main spaces in the body. One space is in the fluid around cells. Another is in the fluid within cells. The third space is in blood.

Fluid balance is the movement of water in and out of these spaces. The sodium in salt moves fluid. If someone sprinkles salt on a slice of potato, water beads on the surface. The sodium draws water out of the plant's cells. The same thing happens in the body.

Sodium controls the flow of water between the three main fluid spaces. At times, sodium levels might be high inside cells. Water from outside the cells moves into the cells. If sodium levels are high outside cells, water moves from the inside of cells to the outside. In general, water follows sodium. That keeps the levels of sodium and water balanced in the body. This movement of fluid brings nutrients into cells. It carries waste out of cells.

THE ROLE OF KIDNEYS

Fluid balance couldn't happen without the kidneys. The kidneys filter sodium from the blood. If there's too much sodium in the blood, the kidneys remove it. The excess sodium passes out of the body through the urine.

The kidneys also balance the body's water levels. If sodium levels are low, the kidneys produce urine high in water content. That lowers the amount of water in the body. Sodium and fluid levels return to balance.

DIGESTION

Salt is important for digestion. The chloride in salt helps break down food in the stomach. The body absorbs nutrients from the digested food. Research suggests that chloride could play a role in regulating the levels of bacteria in the stomach. That helps keep the gut healthy.

FURTHER EVIDENCE

Chapter Two discusses how salt functions in the body. Review the chapter. What is the main point? What is key supporting evidence for that point? The website below provides information on salt. Does the website support an existing piece of evidence in the chapter? Or does it add new information?

KIDS' HEALTH: SALT
abdocorelibrary.com/salt

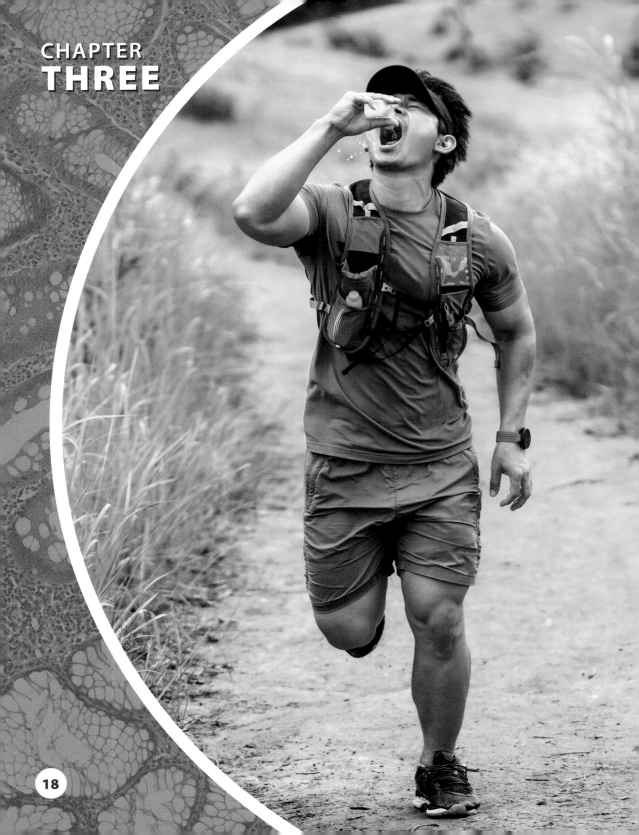

CHAPTER
THREE

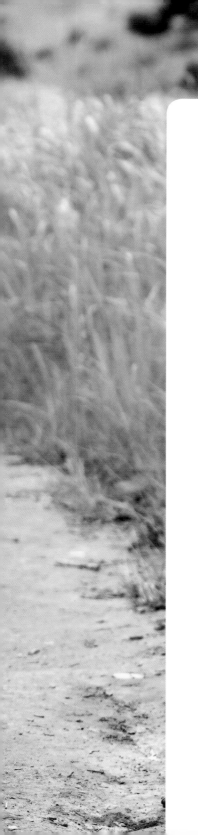

NOT ENOUGH SALT

Most people consume enough salt in a balanced diet. But some people have low levels of sodium. This is called hyponatremia. It can lead to health problems such as dehydration and low blood pressure. Blood pressure is the pressure of blood against the walls of blood vessels.

There are several ways to become low on sodium. People can lose too much sodium if they sweat or urinate a lot. Severe vomiting or diarrhea can result in sodium deficiency. Drinking a lot of water can flush too much

People such as distance runners who exercise for long periods of time are more prone to hyponatremia than others. When they drink, they may not replace enough of the sodium they sweat.

sodium out of the body. Or some people simply don't get enough salt in the foods they eat.

SALT AND EVIL SPIRITS

Have you ever seen people throw salt over their shoulders? That's an old custom from the Middle Ages. People thought it kept demons from sneaking up behind them. Demons were said to dislike salt in their faces. People around the world have believed that evil spirits hate salt. In Japan, salt was sprinkled on stages. People believed it protected the actors from evil spirits. In Haiti, people used salt to break spells. They believed it could make zombies self-aware. In Europe, parents sprinkled salt on or near babies. They did it to protect them from evil.

DEHYDRATION

Lack of salt can lead to dehydration. When sodium passes into cells, it brings water with it. If sodium levels are low, less water moves into cells. The cells become dehydrated.

When people are dehydrated, their skin feels dry. They urinate less. Dehydration can make people feel dizzy and tired. It can make them sick to

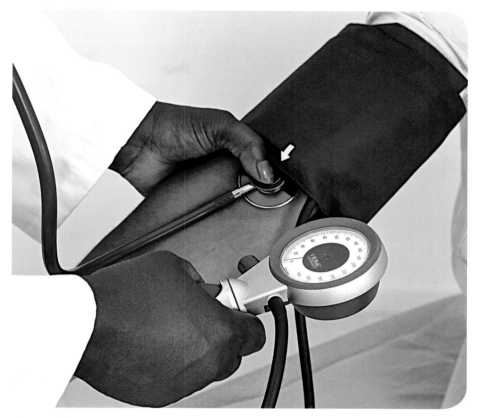

If people are concerned they may have low blood pressure, they can have a doctor check it.

their stomachs. Severe dehydration over long periods can result in serious illness or even death.

LOW BLOOD PRESSURE

Low sodium levels can cause low blood pressure. This is called hypotension. Low blood pressure can lead to dizziness, nausea, and fainting.

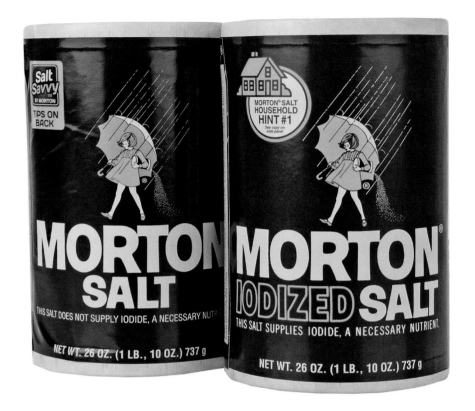

Salt with iodine added to it is called iodized salt.

Sodium is absorbed from the stomach into the blood. Sodium brings water with it into the blood. If sodium is low, fluid levels in blood are low. The volume of the blood is reduced. That results in lower blood pressure. Sodium is one of many factors that control blood pressure.

IODINE

In the United States, most salt is fortified with iodine. Low salt intake can also result in iodine deficiency. Iodine is a mineral. It helps the thyroid function properly. This body part is found in the neck. The thyroid is important for metabolism. Metabolism is the process of converting food into energy. Few foods contain iodine.

IODIZED SALT

Adults low in iodine can get goiters. That's a swelling of the thyroid, which is in the throat. It isn't usually painful. But it can cause a cough. It can make it difficult to breathe and swallow. In the early 1900s, many people in parts of the United States suffered from goiters. The government decided to do something about it. Officials wanted to add iodine to a food that people ate regularly. In 1924, they asked the Morton Salt Company to add iodine to its salt. Iodine is added to salt to this day. Salt with added iodine is called iodized salt.

This is why companies add it to salt. People low in iodine can feel tired and cold. They may gain weight.

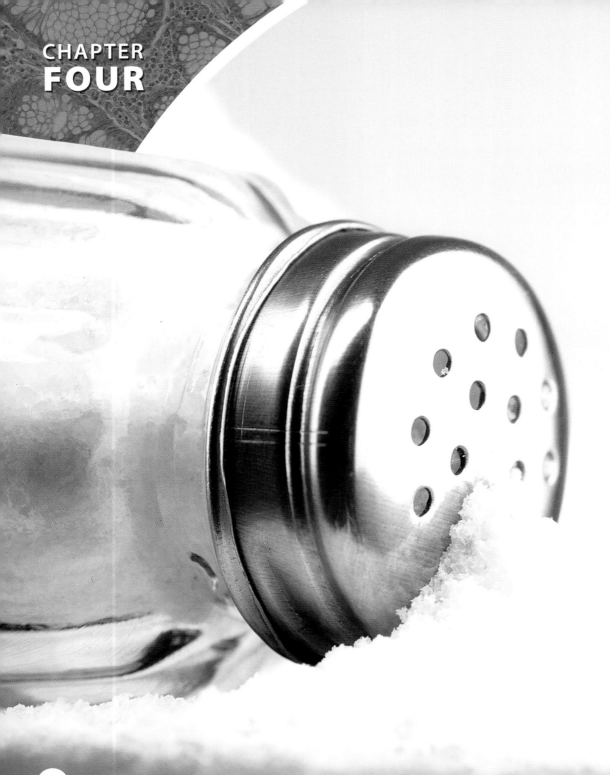

TOO MUCH SALT

Too little salt can be bad for your health. But most people eat plenty of salt. In fact, diets that are too high in salt are more common in the United States. The US Centers for Disease Control and Prevention (CDC) warns that children in the United States eat too much salt every day. A high level of sodium is called hypernatremia. Scientists link it to several health risks.

SWELLING

When the kidneys are healthy, they can handle extra salt. The kidneys filter the extra sodium

Too much salt can cause swelling in certain parts of the body.

out of the blood. They dump it into urine. The excess sodium passes out of the body with the urine.

But if this happens too much, the kidneys can wear out. They have trouble getting rid of the extra sodium. Sodium levels in the blood rise. The body holds on to extra water. It is trying to dilute the sodium.

The extra water gathers in body tissues. This causes swelling. The swelling is called edema. Edema can be painful. Edema can make walking difficult. Blood has a harder time circulating through the body.

OTHER RISKS

Another health risk that is linked to high

ADDICTED TO SALT

You eat one salty chip, then another, and another. It's hard to put the bag down. That's because people naturally enjoy the salty taste. Some studies show that salt releases chemicals in the brain that make people want more. The more people eat salty foods, the more they crave them. That may make it hard for people to reduce salt in their diets if their sodium levels are too high.

KIDNEYS AT WORK

1. High sodium concentration in blood.

5. Sodium concentration in the bloodstream decreases.

2. Pituitary gland releases antidiuretic hormone (ADH).

4. ADH causes water to move from the kidneys back into the bloodstream. There, the water dilutes the sodium.

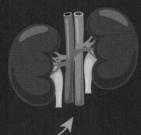

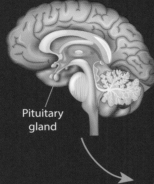

Pituitary gland

3. Blood carries ADH to kidneys.

Hormones tell the kidneys how to balance sodium and water. When sodium levels are high, the body senses the imbalance. It signals the pituitary gland to produce hormones. These hormones are carried by the blood. They travel to the kidneys. The hormones tell the kidneys to conserve water so less is lost through urination. That's why urine tends to be darker yellow if too much salt is consumed. There isn't as much water to dilute it. What would happen if the kidneys couldn't do their job?

salt levels is osteoporosis. That's a condition that causes weak bones. Excess sodium causes the body to absorb more water. So the more salt people eat, the more they have to urinate to get rid of the extra water. Every time

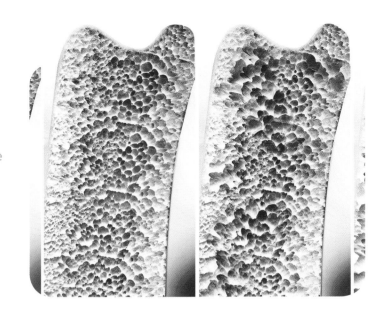

In osteoporosis, the bones gradually get less dense and break more easily.

people urinate, their bodies lose calcium. Calcium is a mineral that builds strong bones. If people urinate too much, their bodies could lose too much calcium. A lack of calcium can result in weak bones and bone loss.

Some studies have shown a link between a high-salt diet and stomach cancer. The connection isn't entirely clear. It may be that too much salt or salt-preserved foods damage the stomach lining. Sores form in the lining. They can become cancerous.

HYPERTENSION

The biggest health risk of a high-salt diet is high blood pressure. The medical term is hypertension. High blood pressure is a leading cause of heart attacks and strokes. More people die from heart attacks and strokes than any other cause in the world. A heart attack happens when blood flow to the heart is blocked. A stroke is when blood flow to an area of the brain is cut off.

Scientists have known about the link between high sodium levels and high blood pressure for many years. But they are not exactly sure how sodium causes high blood pressure. That's because dozens of

WEIGHT LOSS

Scientists did a study on mice in 2017. They found that the more salt the mice ate, the more calories they burned. It appears that a salty diet may help stimulate weight loss, at least in mice. More research will need to be done to see if a human's body responds the same way. Scientists caution against eating more salt to lose weight because of the other health risks it carries.

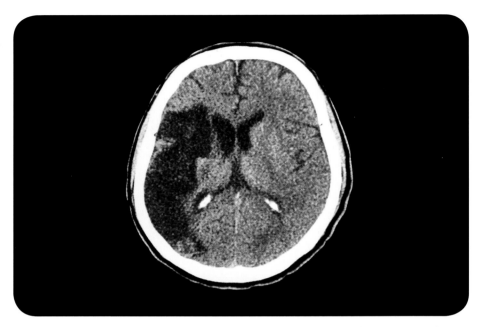

A scan can reveal the damage done to the brain from a stroke, *red area*.

factors in the body help control blood pressure. Diet, exercise, and weight all play a role.

Researchers believe the reason may have to do with how the body reacts to increased fluid in blood. Eating a lot of salt brings extra water into the blood. That increases the volume of blood. That may signal the kidneys to release hormones. The hormones cause blood pressure to rise.

STRAIGHT TO THE
SOURCE

A 2017 article from National Public Radio summarized recent studies that suggest that more salt doesn't always mean more heart disease:

> *Participants in a recent study with the highest intake of sodium and potassium actually had significantly lower blood pressure. . . . The group with the lowest blood pressure averaged a daily sodium intake of 3.7 grams a day, far higher than the guidelines suggest.*
>
> *The findings echo those of a 2016 study published in* The Lancet. *. . . According to the data, moderate to high salt consumption in people with normal blood pressure did not appear to have the dire consequences that might have been presumed.*

Source: Bret Stetka. "Has Salt Gotten an Unfair Shake?" *NPR*. NPR, September 3, 2017. Web. Accessed September 28, 2018.

What's the Big Idea?
Read the primary source text carefully. What is the main idea? Explain how the main idea is supported by details. Name two or three of the supporting details.

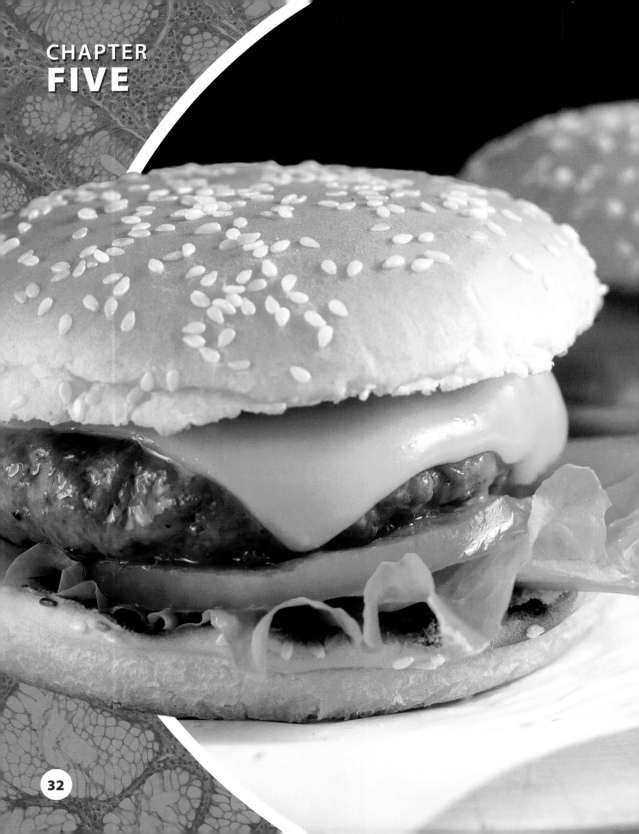

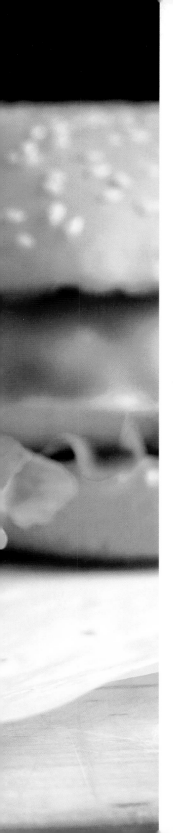

PASS THE SALT OR HIDE THE SHAKER?

S ince the 1970s, doctors and scientists have recommended that people should cut back on salt. Most agree that a low-salt diet can protect against heart disease. The CDC reports that 90 percent of children in the United States eat too much salt every day. One in six children has high blood pressure.

Many adults in the United States will eventually develop high blood pressure. According to one medical report, reducing salt in diets would reduce the number of heart attacks and strokes. This could save as many as 150,000 lives a year just in the United States.

Fast food tends to be high in sodium.

SEA SALT AND TABLE SALT

There are two basic types of salt. They are sea salt and table salt. Both have a similar amount of sodium. The main difference is how they are made. Table salt is usually mined from the ground. It is processed so that it has a uniform, fine texture. Some table salt has iodine added to it. Sea salt comes from oceans or saltwater lakes. It's not processed as much as table salt. It can be fine, coarse, or flaky. It may contain other minerals. However, sea salt is not often fortified with iodine.

But not all experts agree. Some believe that reducing salt doesn't affect blood pressure for most people. Some recent studies suggest that only people with high blood pressure or other health conditions benefit from cutting back on salt.

HOW MUCH IS ENOUGH?

How much salt is enough to stay healthy? How much is too much? Health experts disagree about that too. Some estimate a healthy adult needs approximately 0.7 pounds (0.3 kg) a year. Others estimate more than 15.9 pounds (7.23 kg) a year are needed. Some people need more salt than

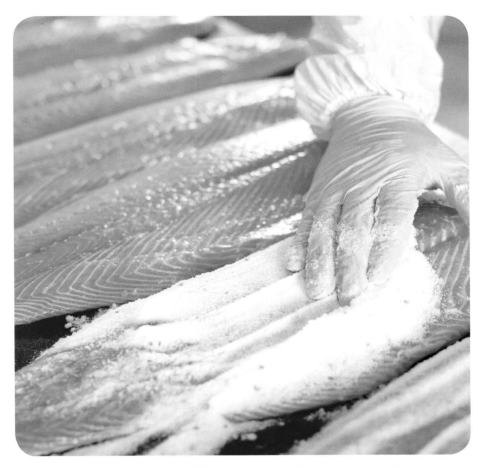

Avoiding foods preserved in or made with a lot of salt is one way to cut back on salt.

others. For example, people who live in hot places and are outdoors a lot sweat more. They need to eat more salt to replace the sodium they lose.

The US government publishes the amount of nutrients it recommends that adults eat based on a

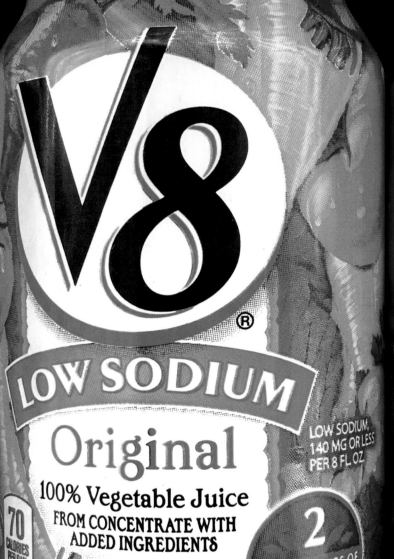

2,000-calorie diet. It calls these amounts the daily values (DVs). The recommended DV for sodium is 2,300 milligrams or less. That's approximately 1 teaspoon of salt.

Some people should eat even less salt. They include people with high blood pressure or close-to-high blood pressure. The US Dietary Guidelines of 2015 recommend these people eat no more than 1,500 milligrams of sodium per day.

SALT SOURCES

Currently, American males eat an average of more than 4,240 milligrams of sodium a day. American females eat an average of more than 2,980 milligrams of sodium a day. Both men and women should be eating no more than 2,300 milligrams a day.

Some people try to cut back on their sodium intake. But it's easy to forget about sodium that naturally occurs

Many foods and beverages come in low-sodium varieties for people who need to cut back on sodium.

in some foods. Red meats such as pork and beef have some salt. Vegetables don't have much salt.

Many people like to add a shake or two of salt to their foods. But the excess salt people consume doesn't come just from saltshakers. Most of it comes from processed foods. Processed foods include canned and frozen foods. Lots of restaurant meals are high in salt too.

Most people like salt and salty foods. Salt is important for good health. Our bodies couldn't function without it. Our bodies can't make sodium, so we must eat salt. But eating too much salt isn't good for us

SOURCES OF SODIUM

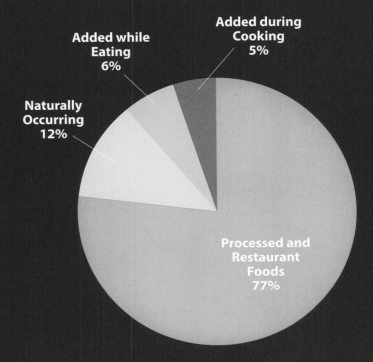

Added during Cooking 5%

Added while Eating 6%

Naturally Occurring 12%

Processed and Restaurant Foods 77%

This chart shows what percentage of sodium Americans get from different foods. Think about your own diet. Based on this chart, do you think you eat the right amount of salt? Or do you eat too much or too little? What could you do to get the right balance of salt?

either. As with all foods, it's important not to consume too much salt. You can use the DV as a guide. Check out the nutrition labels on foods you eat a lot of. See how much sodium they contain. If you have any concerns about salt and your health, talk with your doctor. A little

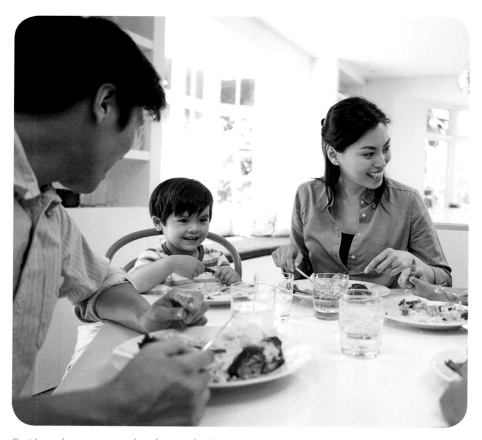

Eating home-cooked meals is a great way to control the amount of salt you eat.

sprinkle of salt now and then can make food tasty and keep your body healthy.

STRAIGHT TO THE
SOURCE

Jane Brody of the *New York Times* makes an argument for reducing salt in the American diet:

> *The overwhelming strength of scientific findings bolsters advice from major health organizations that most Americans should cut back on sodium for the sake of their health. Excess sodium is responsible for most cases of hypertension in Western societies, and hypertension is a leading risk factor for heart attacks and kidney failure.*
>
> *Because salt added to our foods by processors and restaurants, not that from our saltshakers, is the main source of sodium in our diets, protecting the health of the most vulnerable requires a society-wide reduction in sodium.*
>
> Source: Jane Brody. "Clearing Up the Confusion about Salt." *New York Times*. New York Times, November 20, 2017. Web. Accessed September 28, 2018.

Point of View

Compare this excerpt with the one in Chapter Four. What is the point of view of each author? How do they differ in their views on the health risks of salt? Write a short essay comparing the two points of view reflected in the primary sources in this book.

FAST FACTS

- Salt is a natural mineral composed of two elements: sodium (Na) and chloride (Cl). The chemical name of salt is NaCl.

- Dry salt is the only rock that humans eat.

- An average adult's body contains at least 3.5 ounces (100 g) of sodium.

- The sodium and chloride in salt are electrolytes. Electrolytes are minerals that dissolve in body fluids.

- The sodium in salt helps keep body fluids in balance, moves nutrients and oxygen around the body, and helps keep muscles working.

- The chloride in salt aids in digestion.

- Low salt intake can result in dehydration and low blood pressure.

- High salt intake is linked to high blood pressure and heart disease.

- The US government recommends that adults and children eat 2,300 milligrams or less of sodium each day.

- American males eat an average of more than 4,240 milligrams of sodium a day. American females eat an average of more than 2,980 milligrams of sodium a day.

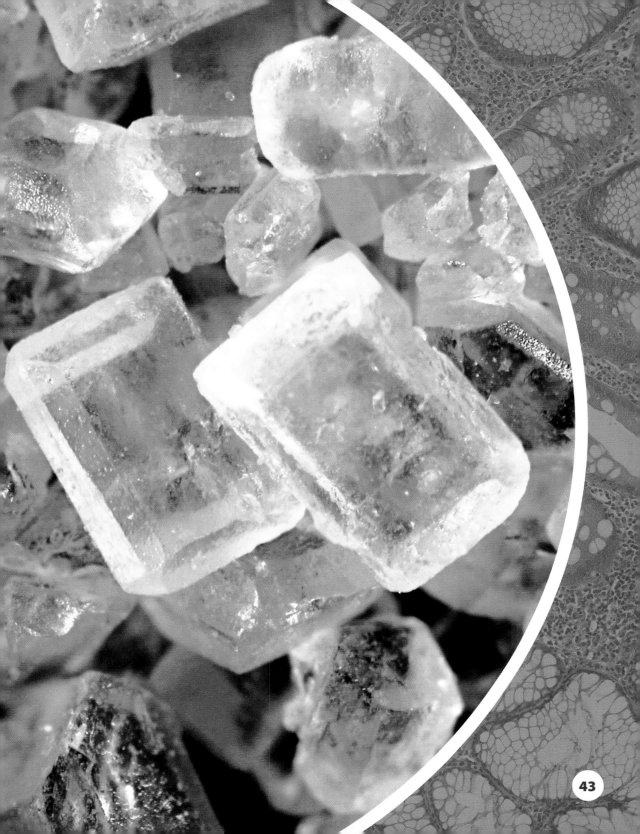

STOP AND
THINK

Tell the Tale

Chapter One of this book describes what happens when someone eats salty popcorn. Imagine you have just eaten a salty snack. How does the salt make you feel? What happens as your body absorbs the salt? Write 200 words about the effect on your body when you eat a lot of salt.

Surprise Me

Chapter Two discusses the function of salt in the body. After reading this chapter, what two or three facts about salt did you find most surprising? Write a few sentences about each fact. Why did you find each fact surprising?

Dig Deeper

After reading this book, what questions do you still have about salt and its effect on your body? With an adult's help, find a few reliable sources that can help you answer your questions. Write a paragraph about what you learned.

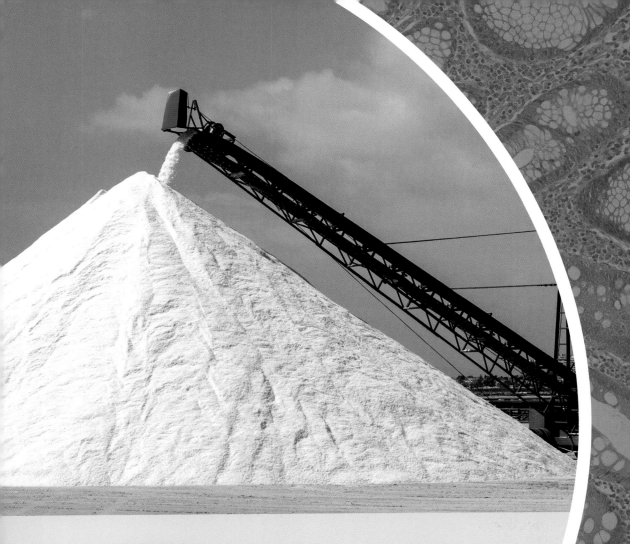

Say What?

Studying salt and nutrition can mean learning a lot of new vocabulary. Find five words in this book you've never heard before. Use a dictionary to find out what they mean. Then write the meanings in your own words, and use each word in a new sentence.

GLOSSARY

cell
the smallest unit of animals and plants that is living and can act on its own

deficiency
the state of lacking something necessary

dehydration
the state of lacking enough water in the body for normal functions

dilute
to make thinner and less concentrated

element
a substance that cannot be divided into smaller units, such as sodium and chloride

gut
stomach or intestines

hormone
a substance made by cells in the body that helps control body processes, such as growth

mined
to have dug underground to get something such as a mineral

pituitary gland
a small gland at the base of the brain that is important in controlling growth and development

processed
having gone through manufacturing

thyroid
a gland in the throat that produces a hormone that regulates growth and the conversion of food to energy

ONLINE RESOURCES

To learn more about your body on salt, visit our free resource websites below.

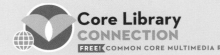

Core Library
CONNECTION
FREE! COMMON CORE MULTIMEDIA RESOURCES

Visit **abdocorelibrary.com** or scan this QR code for free Common Core resources for teachers and students, including vetted activities, multimedia, and booklinks, for deeper subject comprehension.

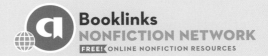

Booklinks
NONFICTION NETWORK
FREE! ONLINE NONFICTION RESOURCES

Visit **abdobooklinks.com** or scan this QR code for free additional online weblinks for further learning. These links are routinely monitored and updated to provide the most current information available.

LEARN MORE

Are You What You Eat? New York: DK Publishing, 2015. Print.

Reinke, Beth Bence. *Nutrition Basics.* Minneapolis, MN: Abdo Publishing, 2016. Print.

INDEX

About the Author

Yvette LaPierre lives in North Dakota with her family, two dogs, and two crested geckos. She writes and edits books and articles for children and adults.